How to Ease Anxiety and Panic Attacks

and

Free Yourself from them

PHILIPPE BRIOUD

TABLE OF CONTENT

Introduction   Pg n°1

Part 1: Some necessary psychological   Pg n°3
considerations

Part 2: Techniques to defuse an attack   Pg n°14
and exercises to prevent one

2.1- Techniques to defuse a panic attack   Pg n°15

2.2- Prevention exercises and lifestyle   Pg n°38
changes

2.2.a- Specific exercises to get through a   Pg n°39
delicate moment

2.2.b- Lifestyle changes   Pg n°60

Part 3: Case study   Pg n°68

Conclusion   Pg n°82

Thank You   Pg n°85

TABLE DES TECHNIQUES DE DESAMORÇAGE

Technique No. 1 : Deep Breathing — Pg n°15

Technique No. 2 : Contracting/Relaxing Muscles — Pg n°18

Technique No. 3 : Stop and Replace — Pg n°19

Technique No. 4 : Drink Plenty of Water — Pg n°21

Technique No. 5 : The 'Cheat Sheet' — Pg n°22

Technique No. 6 : Controlled or Full Breathing — Pg n°24

Technique No. 7 : Find a Distraction — Pg n°27

Technique No. 8 : Go for a Change of Scene — Pg n°30

Technique No. 9 : Seek Solace — Pg n°31

Technique No. 10 : Engage in Physical Activity — Pg n°34

Technique No. 11 : Hyperventilation – Paper Bag Technique or Equivalent — Pg n°35

TABLE DES EXERCICES DE PREVENTION

Exercise No. 1 : Abdominal Breathing — Pg n°39

Exercise No. 2 : Complete Breathing — Pg n°40

Exercise No. 3 : Visualize Calm — Pg n°41

Exercise No. 4 : Chanting a Mantra — Pg n°42

Exercise No. 5 : Get out of your Comfort Zone — Pg n°43

Exercise No. 6 : Rationalize your Overall Anxiety — Pg n°46

Exercise No. 7 : Make Time for Free Anxiety — Pg n°47

Exercise No. 8 : Let Everything Explode — Pg n°48

Exercise No. 9 : Ask Yourself Whether the Problem Can Be Solved — Pg n°51

Exercise No. 10 : Watch a Comedy — Pg n°53

Exercise No. 11 : Keep a Private Journal — Pg n°54

Exercise No. 12 : Choose the Things You Wish to See — Pg n°55

Exercise No. 13 : Make Love More Often   Pg n°56

Exercise No. 14 : Make a Clean Sweep   Pg n°56

Exercise No. 15 : Go for a Walk in the Woods   Pg n°58

Exercise No. 16 : So, Then ? How About that Half-full Glass ?   Pg n°58

INTRODUCTION

Anxiety is an everyday problem for more and more people. Sometimes it may lead to actual panic attacks. I, myself, experienced them for about two years of my life. I know the vicious circle that gradually builds in the life of the anxious person. I also know how to escape from it, and this is what I want to share in this book.

Know that it's possible to overcome this disability and to live with panic attacks. However, if the attacks occur frequently, and are debilitating, I advise you to get cognitive behavioral therapy. Nevertheless, if they are happening because of a stressful situation in your adult life, the panic attacks are likely to be temporary and completely reversible. This book will help you find the serenity to deal with anxious situations and teach you how to handle them calmly, without panic.

In Part 1, we discuss certain psychological considerations that contribute to the condition of the anxious person. These may be anything from a negative social situation to the efforts needed to break free of it. Then, in Part 2, we examine several techniques to defuse a nascent anxiety attack as well as preventative exercises and essential lifestyle principles which help reduce anxiety in daily life. Finally, in Part 3, we take a deeper look at the evolution of a panic attack by means of a case study in order to expand our knowledge of visualization techniques and how to make best use of the solutions recommended in this book when a dreaded panic attack strikes.

I hope you enjoy reading this book, and take heart, because I know that living with anxiety attacks can be very difficult.

PART 1:
SOME NECESSARY PSYCHOLOGICAL CONSIDERATIONS

If you bought this book, it's either because you are plagued with panic attacks, or someone dear to you is. Therefore, I won't go into a detailed description of the physical sensations that one can experience during an attack, as you know them all too well, the free press writes about them all the time, and that's enough of that. At best, it will reassure you to know that when you feel as if you are choking, like you are going to pass out or perhaps even die, that it's entirely normal to feel this way during a panic attack. Therefore, it is better that we focus on the psychological dimension without playing the role of psychotherapist.

Anxiety is often linked to a type of neurotic or

psychotic disorder. We can easily say that there is a tendency towards seeing the glass half-empty rather than half-full. This pessimistic attitude cannot be changed overnight. Maybe you flat-out refuse to change it as it constitutes a principle for you in life. Allow me, then, to try and make you reconsider this outlook; doing so will go a long ways towards eliminating your panic attacks and will help you live a happier, healthier life.

If you can only see the glass as half-empty, it's possible that you were never shown an alternative way of thinking. Let's stop to observe certain situations from two different points of view :

- "I missed my bus. I'll be even later than I already am. My boss will reprimand me; maybe he'll even fire me !" OR "I missed my bus. I'll be able to finish this chapter of my book, or listen to this song that I really like while I wait for the next one. I'll take the opportunity to relax a bit; I'll be extra productive this morning and I'll still look good. At worst, I'll leave work a little later tonight."

- "I broke my shoe. Next time it rains, it will get wet and it's obvious that it's busted. Oh, why do these things always happen to me !" OR "I broke my shoe. My friends will laugh when I tell them the story. Perhaps they'll recommend a new store with excellent and beautiful shoes."

- "I haven't heard from my boyfriend. Maybe something happened to him, or he's cheating on me with somebody else. Men, they're all scoundrels !" OR "I haven't heard from my boyfriend. Traffic must be bad, or perhaps he stopped to buy me flowers. No, couldn't be, he never does that ! He must be stuck in traffic."

- "This baby's ears look like cauliflower. It will be ugly later." OR "This baby's ears look like cauliflower, but he has such beautiful eyes. Hopefully, his ears will look better as he gets older."

Note that the final conclusions drawn by each point of view are radically different. However, the sentences themselves are not very different, or at least they both begin the same way regardless of whether the outlook is pessimistic or more positive.

Quite often, we tell people who see the glass half-full that they are a bit silly. If that's what you think, re-examine the previous examples, and you will see that it is just not true.

Many times, we want to know who is wrong and who is right. This is wrong because that's not the issue. Especially since the person who sees the glass half-empty often sees things in the realm of the hypothetical, and this leads him to make generalizations that will eventually be proven false. In reality, it's just an outlook or angle of observation. It can't be helped, it is what it is, and that's how it goes. (Once again, a defeatist attitude.) In reality, it is quite possible to move away from this mode of thinking, but it requires some effort.

And, if you say that life ain't easy, and it won't be that way anytime soon, note that this is another way of seeing the glass half-empty and of making assumptions on what the future will bring. I sincerely believe that if this is the way you think, you are right. Yes, you are right; life ain't easy ... as far as you're concerned. In fact, even when life is good to you, you'll never notice because you (unconsciously) reject seeing the glass half-full.

Therefore, in the future, try not to speak too soon. See if it's not possible to view the current situation differently. There is a way to see things differently, and much more optimistically, without looking silly. It's up to you to make the effort. To help you, here is a quote from Marcus Aurelius : **"Our life is what our thoughts make it."** It's all summed up in this quote. Take the time to read it again. Write it down and put it somewhere where you can be reminded of it every day, perhaps a daily reminder on your cell phone (memo), or a post-it note stuck to the bathroom mirror.

To help you work on changing your thoughts, here are a few cognitive distortions that you **must stop now** :

- **Generalization** : Making generalizations based on a single negative experience. For example : "I messed up this interview, I'll flub them all and I'll never find a job." Or "I had a panic attack at the restaurant this afternoon. I should never go to restaurants for lunch because I'll have a panic attack every time." This is obviously counter-productive.

- **Exaggerated ideas** : When you see things as black and white, with no half measures. For example : "I had a panic attack this afternoon, I'm such a loser !" or "If my boss criticizes me over this job, my career is ruined !"

- **Mental filter** : Focusing on negative events and being blind to the positive. For example : "She always says bad things about me.", which is not necessarily true. Or "I have a panic attack every time I drive this route."; without taking into consideration that you were trying to parallel park in downtown Paris without getting blasted by the horns of other motorists.

- **Mitigating the positive** : For example, "I got this contract, but it's only dumb luck." Just maybe it was because you did a good job. This, then, had nothing to do with luck, but with your sweat, your thoughts and your actions.

- **Predicting the future** : This is when you imagine negative outcomes that are not based on any real element. For example : "I don't know why, but something feels wrong." Even if you are a very intuitive person, your intuition can sometimes be wrong. Don't take a defeatist attitude; this will only attract more disappointments.

- **Doom-mongering** : Expecting the worst case scenario in every situation. For example : "The road is narrow and we need to drive near the ravine, we'll fall for sure."

- **Labeling** : For example : "I'm a loser." Or "I'm an idiot." There is no need to insult yourself even if you did make a mistake. Always respect yourself.

- **Emotional deduction** : For example, "I'm afraid, so it'll never work." Managing your emotions is something that can be very difficult. Start by noticing the times when your emotions lead you to negative inferences or exaggerated apprehension.

- **Taking things personally** : Assuming responsibility for things that are beyond your control. For example, "It's my fault my husband cheated on me." Or "My friend was coming to get me when she crashed into the truck, so her accident is all my fault."

All these ways of thinking are obviously very toxic, and can make you anxious. Maybe you don't realize you have these types of thoughts sometimes. **Learn to identify and reformulate your ideas in a more realistic manner**.

Now, let's get back to our panic attacks.

What is a panic attack from a physiological point of view? It's an exaggerated response of the brain, which believes it is facing a dangerous situation, so it triggers the fight or flight response. This mechanism dates from the time when our ancestors lived in caves and may have needed to run away to escape a ferocious beast at a moment's notice. Fortunately, the context of life has changed since then, but not the functioning of our brain.

Now, when faced with an anxiety-producing situation, such as the fear of not being good enough or the anxiety felt when you attempt to suppress your emotions, you try to gain control over your feelings. Unfortunately, the result is that your brain reinforces these warning signals because you seem oblivious to the danger. The more you try to repress these feelings, perhaps to impress the people you're with, or even when you're alone, the more your brain will reinforce them. **This is the downward spiral of a panic attack**. A kind of ping-pong between you and your body (brain) with each episode being more intense than the last.

Therefore, it is best to **accept the situation**. It is perfectly normal to be anxious when facing certain situations (meeting with the boss to explain a delay, negotiations with a bank to obtain a loan, a tryst, etc.). In other situations, it may not seem normal to be anxious (getting up in the morning or going to bed at night, driving a car, eating out with friends, etc.). However, if you have a profile that favors negativity and if you have had panic attacks in the past, it's not so unusual that **anticipatory anxiety** may be a problem for you. This is where the vicious cycle traps you, causing you to limit your social interactions and do little more than remain cloistered at home (safe).

For more information about anticipatory anxiety, please refer to the beginning of this chapter where we explore various aspects about seeing the glass half-empty versus half-full. It might be a good idea to read this part again once you've read the entire book because changing bad habits and thoughts is not an easy task, and can't be done on demand. Logically, you may believe that these fears are not justified. However, this is not enough to break the vicious circle of anxiety.

And, above all, don't try to avoid anxious situations to alleviate anticipatory anxiety. Having a meal with friends when some of the guests are unknown to you may create an anxiety-producing situation where you get the urge to escape by canceling at the last minute. If this is the case, YOU MUST GO. And you'll find that it won't kill you. A maxim to remember is : **"What we fear the most is what we most need to do."** When you find yourself in the vicious circle of anxiety, remember this.

Before concluding this first part, I want to emphasize that you should never feel shameful about experiencing panic attacks. Studies indicate that about one in every five people will experience an attack at least once in their lives. Think about ten people you know, two of them are either having or have had panic attacks in the past. So, if you're one of them, don't feel you have to go into hiding. This doesn't mean that you need to broadcast to the world the fact that you suffer this type of problem. Just accept it, and understand that it's not completely abnormal for someone to feel this way. And, among those ten people who you thought about previously, at least two are affected by anxiety, and perhaps three others may be afflicted by more serious issues, even though you may not be aware of it. Above all, don't blame yourself or feel shame for your panic attacks; many have, or have had, or will have panic attacks. Don't waste your time and energy worrying about it, it is what it is. Just accept it, and take yourself in hand, because it is possible to return to a life that is more 'normal' and more serene.

The second part of this book teaches you various techniques and exercises to help prevent the onset and escalation of panic attacks. Are you game ? Yes ? Then let's continue.

Things to take away from Part 1 :

- Take the view that the glass is half-full rather than half-empty. It is not silly to have a positive attitude.

"Our life is what our thoughts make it."

- The brain sometimes sends exaggerated danger signals.

- Don't try to avoid anxiety-provoking situations to alleviate anticipatory anxiety. "What we fear the most is what we most need to do."

- Shame doesn't need to add your current difficulties.

PART 2:
TECHNIQUES TO DEFUSE AN ATTACK
AND EXERCISES TO PREVENT ONE

In this chapter, I will outline a series of defusion techniques to use when a panic attack strikes. This will be followed by a number of preventative exercises that will help reduce the frequency of these attacks, perhaps even eliminate them from your life altogether.

Among all these techniques, there are some you will find more appealing than others. Try them all. Then, continue using the ones that work best for you. You'll discover that, depending on the situation, there are times you may prefer one technique over another. Therefore, keep several of these techniques in mind, or even all of them, because they all may serve you sooner or later.

2. 1- TECHNIQUES TO DEFUSE A PANIC ATTACK

First of all, remember that the battle is lost ahead of time. When you feel the first symptoms of an attack, the more you fight against it, the stronger it gets. Therefore, accept it for what it is. When it starts, notice what is happening and use the following techniques before the symptoms escalate. At first, you may not notice much effect. In fact, don't even try to see any effect. Simply administer the technique **by focusing on applying the steps below in the best possible manner**. Later in the day, you can remind yourself of that earlier moment when you successfully averted a panic attack.

At the onset of an attack :

Technique No. 1 : Deep Breathing

You feel your level of anxiety mounting. Of course, you have no idea why, it seems to come out of nowhere. What is certain is that an attack is coming. When this happens, **breathe deeply**, and **focus** on this breathing.

- Start by inhaling through the nose for three to four seconds.

- Hold your breath for three to four seconds.

- Exhale through the mouth, slowly, for three to four seconds in much the same way that you would blow on hot food to cool it off. The exhale should be a little forced, and the lips should be pursed to channel the air coming out of your mouth.

Breathe in this manner for a few minutes. Two to three minutes should be enough to cause all symptoms of anxiety to disappear, to be replaced with a sense of relaxation and well-being. If it takes a little longer for you to calm down, just keep practicing this technique for as long as it takes.

The important thing to keep in mind in order to ensure the effectiveness of this technique, as well as that of the other techniques that follow, is to stop focusing on the symptoms of the attack. Instead, keep your mind on practicing the technique to the best of your ability. Don't stop after a minute or two to check if the symptoms are dissipating because the very act of focusing on them is the best way to find them, even if they are not really there. This is part of the paradox of the panic attack; it tends to bring out our tendencies towards hypochondria. We quickly find something that's not going well only to return to the escalating torment of an attack. Instead, **just focus on practicing the technique in the proper manner**.

Tip : To obtain a better focus on your breathing, use a sharp, refreshing and strong-smelling scent such as facial tissues with a eucalyptus scent, mint-flavored chewing gum or strong breath mints, or pure lavender essential oil mixed with water and sprayed onto a handkerchief. However, avoid hard candies that are of average size and difficult to break because these may trigger the fear of choking.

The idea here is to spread a feeling of freshness in our lungs. This reduces the sensation that you're having breathing difficulties and helps increase the calming aspect of deep breathing.

Another technique which may lack the freshness, but is more soothing, is to use a piece of cloth which carries the scent of someone who is dear to you.

Technique No. 2 : Contracting/Relaxing Muscles

This technique involves creating artificial muscle tension that will later resolve into muscle relaxation. The latter will cause overall relaxation of your body and your mind.

To do this, we will first force our muscles to tense and then suddenly release the tension. The reason for this is twofold : it causes you to consume and channel your flagging energy, and promotes the relaxation effect during the second stage.

Step #1 - muscle tension : **Clench your fists tightly** for three to four seconds. This contracts the muscles in your arms. You can also stretch out your legs while pointing your toes (do this while sitting in a chair or lying on a bed). This will contract the muscles in your thighs and calves as well as your abdominals.

Step #2 - muscle relaxation : **Suddenly release** the muscle tension that was applied in Step #1, **while simultaneously expelling all the air** from your lungs. This will cause you to take a deep breath afterwards. This feeling of relaxation flows naturally throughout your body, and the full exhalation eliminates toxins from your blood. Combined with a deep inhalation, your blood and your organs, including the brain, are cleansed and refreshed through the process of oxygenation.

By focusing intently on the process, practicing this technique for two to three minutes will get you in tune with the **present moment**. From this point on, you can approach the situation **more calmly**.

However, be careful. If you experience any pain or tingling in your muscles, don't force it and move to another technique.

Another word of warning, do not use your facial muscles for Step #1, especially not your jaw, as doing this would produce the opposite effect and intensify the feeling of nausea. It is always best to keep your facial muscles relaxed.

Technique No. 3 : Stop and Replace

This technique requires a certain amount of mental ability or discipline. It can be difficult for some people to achieve. A regular meditation practice can be a great help in mastering this technique.

You feel the symptoms of the panic attack coming on and say to yourself, "That's it, there I go again, I can't escape, I'll fall apart !" or other agonizing thoughts along those lines. The "stop and replace" technique can help you get out of this negative state of mind, and stave off the still-emerging panic attack. It is important to remember that your mindset has a great influence the intensity and duration of an attack.

The technique consists of literally stopping the agonizing thoughts and replacing them with calmer, more peaceful ones. For example, when anxious thoughts begin to take more and more room in your mind, just say **"Stop !"** and **replace them** with other ideas such as : "When is my next night out with the girls ?" OR "Why not go on a little romantic holiday in the countryside or by the beach this weekend ?" OR "What shall I give my sister for her birthday present ?" OR "I think I'll go for a bike ride, where will I go this time ?" I think you understand the concept. Thinking in this manner will calm your thoughts and direct your attention towards **more joyful** events. Immerse yourself in these new thoughts and use them to break away from the downward spiral. It will do you good.

I know that this can sometimes be difficult to achieve. Once again, practicing meditation regularly can change the score. We'll go into more in detail about this in the chapter on best lifestyle practices.

Tip : This is similar to what was discussed in Part 1, but instead of simply telling yourself to stop **worrying in the here and now**, make an effort to imagine yourself **happy or calm elsewhere in the not-too-distant future**. Take a break from all the negativity and devise a plan to enjoy future activities.

Technique No. 4 : Drink Plenty of Water

The simple act of drinking water will refresh your palate, and will make your breath more pleasant and deeper at the same time.

The very act of **being well-hydrated** eliminates many symptoms of anxiety, such as dry mouth, knots in the throat, nausea, etc.

Drinking several glasses of water is the best way rehydrate after the heavy sweating and fatigue that occur during a panic attack.

Finally, **your attention becomes focused** on the act of drinking. Noticing the fresh water gently passing through your mouth and making its way to your stomach will produce a **significantly pleasant distraction**. It is not much, I agree, but it can be effective when coupled with other distractions. Later, we will examine another technique based on distraction.

If you have difficulty swallowing, place a finger at the level of the trachea, just above your rib cage. When you apply a small amount of pressure to this area, **swallowing becomes easier**.

I don't recommend eating dry food during a panic attack, as you may have difficulty swallowing, or may even experience a choking sensation. Therefore, if an attack strikes while you're eating, stop immediately and drink a large glass of water as this will help with the symptoms. Enjoy it as long as your sense of clarity is present.

Technique No. 5 : The 'Cheat Sheet'

This technique is useful at the start of an attack, when you start to get that feeling that something isn't quite right, although you can't figure out just what. **Before going any further, take out your 'cheat sheet'.**

You understand the basic principle of a 'cheat

sheet'; it provides the correct answers. Used in this context, the goal is to find the **right answers** by asking the **right questions**. The idea is to think logically rather than emotionally.

The more comprehensive the 'cheat sheet', the more effective it will be.

Here are a few examples of questions (or answers) to include in your 'cheat sheet' :

- Is there really a good reason to believe that something is wrong ?

- What proof do I have that something is wrong ?

- Could I be exaggerating the situation ?

- This is a problem, not a catastrophe.

- This is just a difficult time, it won't last forever.

Always carry this 'cheat sheet' around with you. You can read it every day as a reminder until you eventually start coming up with the right answers before the problems even present themselves (a useful technique you can also teach your children).

Create this 'cheat sheet' during a calm period, when all is quiet. Now, bring to mind the moments when you were experiencing a panic attack. Think about which thoughts would have been helpful to you during the attack and list them on a sheet of paper (or perhaps a piece of cardboard so it will last longer). **Make your own personal 'cheat sheet'.** To keep with this analogy, when faced with exams, different students are unlikely to list the same items on their 'cheat sheet' as each student has his or her own strengths and weaknesses. This is why, for this technique to be effective, you must make your own personal 'cheat sheet'.

Technique No. 6 : Controlled or Full Breathing

More intense than the "deep breathing" technique mentioned previously, we have the "controlled" or "complete" breathing technique.

Personally, I prefer the term "complete" because it implies, of course, that we usually practice incomplete breathing. For example, it is likely that while you are reading this book, with each inhalation you replace a scant thirty per cent of the volume of air in your lungs. This feeling of not getting enough air is one of the symptoms of an anxiety attack, as you probably know quite well.

However, the term "controlled" is accurate as well. Indeed, it will be necessary to make an effort to breathe in this manner. But don't worry, anybody can do it.

In practical terms, the technique consists of **completely filling the lungs** (the bottom, the middle, and the top). The bottom part of the lungs is filled by practicing abdominal or "belly" breathing. To do this, we use the belly, or more specifically the diaphragm (big muscle under the lungs). The middle of the lungs is filled by thoracic breathing which properly opens the lungs and the ribcage. Finally, the top portion of the lungs is filled by clavicular breathing, a method in which the shoulders are raised slightly to allow air to stay in the upper part of the lungs.

The complete controlled or full breathing technique is the sum of these three types of breathing (abdominal, thoracic and clavicular).

To practice a complete breath, begin by slightly inflating the belly. This has the effect of shifting your diaphragm and releasing air from the lower portion of your lungs. Inhale and when you feel as though the bottom part of the lungs is full, gradually allow the oxygen to flow towards the middle part of the lungs. Open up your chest and allow your ribcage to expand until you feel that the lungs are filled to capacity. At this point, you can accommodate more air at the top of your lungs by lifting your shoulders slightly.

Once your lungs are completely filled, hold the breath for three to four seconds. Don't worry about a slight sensation of dizziness, it is only temporary and disappears once you start exhaling.

Then, exhale the air by gently performing the movement in reverse order. Start by releasing the air at the top of your lungs. Your shoulders drop slightly. Then, slowly deflate your rib cage and allow it to close. Finally, expel the air from the bottom of your lungs by pulling in the belly slightly so as to cause the diaphragm to move up. It is this final motion which dislodges the remaining air from the bottom of the lungs.

The exhalation must last slightly longer than the inhalation.

This complete breathing technique can be practiced while lying down, while sitting or while standing. The back must be straight. It is best to breathe through the nose as this will facilitate control of this respiratory movement.

This technique is also one of the preventative exercises that are examined in the next chapter. In fact, when practiced regularly, it can help you relax on a daily basis. However, it is important to perform this technique properly so that you are comfortable with it in the event that you need to use it to deal with a panic attack.

To defuse an attack, take several breaths in this manner. Be sure to keep your focus exclusively on your breathing for a few minutes until you successfully circumvent the onset of an attack.

Once again, remember not to check if it "works". **You just need to focus on performing the technique and forget about the rest to ensure its success.**

Technique No. 7 : Find a Distraction

When we feel an attack coming on, and the symptoms are getting worse, we tend to make the mistake of focusing on the symptoms. As you know, this only makes them worse. Nevertheless, it is no simple matter to divert our attention at such a moment, hence, the importance of the following technique.

The main idea here is to distract yourself or, to be more specific, **to distract your mind**. Take charge and force yourself to concentrate on other things; it will stimulate your mind to the point that you'll be able to gain control over your thinking. To learn how to do this, let's learn more about our brain's capabilities.

The human brain can focus on about seven elements simultaneously. This means that, during a panic attack, focusing on the paint color of a wall in the room won't help much as you still have enough brain power to think about that horrible, nauseating feeling that's currently threatening to overwhelm you.

Therefore, you need to find a more absorbing distraction. If you are with other people, the ideal thing would be to re-enter a conversation and try to be a relevant part of it.

Unfortunately, if you are unable to speak, or if you happen to be alone at the time, you need to find something else. Here are a few examples :

- If you cannot speak, pay close attention to the conversations around you.

- Say the recipe for your favorite dish out loud and visualize yourself preparing it for people you love.

- Prepare your shopping list : what is missing from the fridge ?

- Recite a poem you know well, a prayer if you are religious, or even a song. Concentrate on the deeper meaning of the verses.

- Count the white hairs on the cat or dog sitting next to you, or in the beard of a man close by.

- Count the number of red cars driving by and try to determine where they come from so you can figure out which area buys red cars the most.

- Recite the letters of the alphabet backwards.

Any distraction **should keep you busy for at least a few minutes** before you have a chance to think of doing something else. This prevents your brain from thinking about your symptoms and realizing that there could be a good (bad) reason to send out alert signals. You can also combine distractions. In moments like these, be inventive !

What to do when a panic attack is already well underway :

We are in the midst of the worst part of the attack. Small, gentle techniques won't do the trick when symptoms are at their peak. At this point, it is no longer a question of averting an attack; we now need to contend with the current situation. However, the following techniques can drastically reduce the intensity of a panic attack and help resolve it.

Technique No. 8 : Go for a Change of Scene

If an attack is already well underway, but you are still able to move, then **change your surroundings**. If you are in a building, go outside, get some fresh air and go for a walk. If you are already outside, look for a change of scene. Walk down the road to the park, or if you're already in the park, change seats and sit on another bench. Or just go home. If you are in a house, go to another room.

If you are at home, and are able to do so, try changing the soundscape. Put on some relaxing music or simply switch to another radio station.

A change of scene is a new situation. Your brain will adapt to its new surroundings; it's a form of distraction for it. This relates to the principle on which the distraction technique is based. Hence, it could be more soothing to "take risks", for example, go for a walk in an unfamiliar park or take a different route home. The idea is to get out of your comfort zone, and while doing so, seeing something new. This doesn't mean getting lost in the forest or taking a stroll in an unsafe neighborhood. **Just change your surroundings; your brain will do the rest**.

Technique No. 9 : Seek Solace

Ask a friend for help. When a panic attack is threatening to overwhelm you, confide in a friend or, at the very least, a trusted person who is aware of your unexpected attacks.

If an attack should arise, your friend needs to learn

this technique. Therefore, assuming you are a woman and your friend is as well, ask her to read the following as this is what she needs to know or do (I will address it directly to her) :

- Be patient. Do not put pressure on your friend to "get over" her attack as it won't last long.

- Reassure your friend and take her by the hand as this will help bring her back to reality. The contact should be strong, powerful and calming, while remaining light and respectful. Do not hold your friend in your arms too tightly unless she has asked you to, as she needs to breathe.

- Do not leave her alone. If you have water, this is perfect, as your friend will need some. If not, go find some with her, but do not abandon her.

- Placing a damp handkerchief on her face will help with nausea and hot flashes, but only do so with your friend's permission.

- If it's possible to go out and get some fresh air together, do so.

- Avoid the presence of other people as this will make your friend feel uncomfortable. See if you can find a calm place away from the stares of other people.

- Encourage your friend to take deep breaths. Help her along by demonstrating how. At times like these, it is difficult for her to control her breathing.

- From time to time, ask her how she is doing. If she cannot stop apologizing for the situation, smile, tell her not to worry and that this is what friends are for. This will go a long way towards helping her to calm down and feel at ease.

- Help her imagine a happy resolution to this situation. "That's better. You're breathing calmly. You're coming back. Don't worry, nobody will ask about what happened. Let's just be calm, it's lunchtime, so let's have a picnic outside in the sunshine. What do you say ? What would you like to eat ?" I think you get the idea.
If there's nobody around that you feel you can trust during an attack, you could phone a close friend or family member. The problem here is you can't be sure that they're available and, if they are, you'll likely take up a good few minutes of their time.

A variation consists of using a technique in which you play a soothing and gentle message from a person close to you. If you're having difficulty contacting the person, or are waiting for them to reply to your message, this technique can reassure you and help you to think of something else.

Forget about emails or instant messages as these are not worth it. Written words are often difficult to interpret and may even be considered a nuisance. Listening to a **person's voice**, either face-to-face or over the phone is a thousand times more pleasant and effective in helping you through these awful moments. Because of its intonation, a voice is something that can't be replaced by writing.

Technique No. 10 : Engage in Physical Activity

When a panic attack strikes, it produces a strong reaction in your brain, which becomes convinced that the body is in a dangerous situation. This will trigger a phenomenon known as the **fight** or **flight** response. In either of these two possible outcomes, the body must exert a substantial physical effort. Therefore, your brain secretes a burst of hormones to help you do battle or flee from the perceived danger. Unfortunately, if you don't "use up" these hormones, they will feed your level of anxiety.

Of course, the level of activity that you are able to engage in will depend on where you happen to be at the time. It is up to you to adapt to the situation. Find something to do which demands a bit of energy consumption by **working your muscles**.

If you are at home, you can do some housework. If you are at the office, you can tidy up your work space, straighten out the files in your cabinet or go look for a new notebook. Take the stairs and run up each one. If you are outside, you could improvise a little; do a bit of jogging, some flex-extension exercises, or some weightlifting. Again, a lot depends on your circumstances, but you have everything to gain when engaging in physical activity.

Specific case :

Technique No. 11 : Hyperventilation – Paper Bag Technique or Equivalent

Sometimes, during a panic attack, hyperventilation can occur. This is short and rapid breathing due to an imbalance between levels of oxygen (O_2) and carbon dioxide (CO_2) in the blood. The respiration rate is based on the level of carbon dioxide in the blood. During hyperventilation, the level of carbon dioxide is lower than normal. The body interprets this as a respiratory problem, which results in hyperventilation. Therefore, it's a vicious circle you need to escape from.

One technique to re-establish adequate levels of carbon dioxide and resume normal respiration consists of breathing into a paper bag. Please do not use a plastic bag as it is dangerous and could completely obstruct your respiratory system.

You only need to breathe into the paper bag a few times. The carbon dioxide level in your blood will rise and the hyperventilation will decrease.

It's not necessary to always have a paper bag on hand, simply take your hands and place them around the nose and mouth while breathing in and out a few times. This works in more or less the same way as using a paper bag, is safer, and you do not need to carry a paper bag around.

Only use this technique during an episode of hyperventilation, and then only to calm it down. However, a panic attack can continue even after the hyperventilation subsides. Since this technique does not calm a panic attack, it is of no use when there is no hyperventilation. On the contrary, a little more oxygen won't hurt. The best thing to do is to go outside and get some fresh air.

This is the end of the defusion techniques. Read them over from time to time, memorize them and think on them if need be.

Let's move on and examine various preventative exercises which can be integrated into your life to improve your anxiety levels and reduce the number of panic attacks.

2.2- PREVENTION EXERCISES AND LIFESTYLE CHANGES

2.2.A- SPECIFIC EXERCISES TO GET THROUGH A DELICATE MOMENT

Exercise No. 1 : Abdominal Breathing

The aim of this exercise is to reduce your overall level of anxiety through better breathing. Practicing good breathing is the foundation of a number of meditation techniques, and with good reason as it effectively reduces tension in the body. By practicing deep breathing techniques, our parasympathetic system (responsible for relaxation of the body) gains control over the sympathetic system (responsible for alert triggers).

Most adults breathe thoracically, which makes use of only thirty percent of the lungs' capacity. However, a nursing infant breathes abdominally and uses seventy percent.

This difference in volume is due to the fact that with thoracic breathing, we only use the top portion of the lungs, while with abdominal breathing, we also fill up the lower part.

Practicing abdominal breathing is very easy. Start by exhaling while lightly pulling in the lower part of the abdomen. This will enable you to empty out your lungs completely. A deeper inhalation will naturally follow. Your abdomen will inflate a little, but not so much that becomes distended. Then, exhale again while lightly pulling in your abdomen. It's simple and almost too easy. Breathing in this manner is a great way to reduce your anxiety levels. To ensure that each inhalation and exhalation lasts a few seconds, count up to five or six in your head, depending on how intense you want the exercise to be.

Practice this exercise several times a day, whenever you have a few minutes to spare. It is very simple and discreet, and you can do it anytime : while waiting for public transport as well as in your car at a red light. You'll find that your anxiety levels will be greatly reduced over the course of the day.

Exercise No. 2 : Complete Breathing

As you will probably have guessed, complete breathing is an extension of the previous exercise.

In this exercise, the volume of air taken in by your lungs is close to one hundred percent. This exercise forms part of the aforementioned techniques to help you to defuse a panic attack. This was already explained and I refer you to that section so that you can learn more about it and practice it (Technique n°7 : complete or controlled breathing).

I list the exercise again here as it can be used as an exercise to reduce daily anxiety. This method of breathing is somewhat less discreet than abdominal breathing, and ideally it should be practiced in a peaceful and private place. Spend at least ten minutes a day for two or three weeks so that you **master it and know how to use it as a defusion technique**.

Exercise No. 3 : Visualize Calm

This exercise can be likened to a light meditation. It consists of visualizing a calm, relaxing scene, and otherwise emptying your mind. It can be compared to perhaps gazing into a blue sky or watching water flow slowly by.

For a few minutes, switch off the phone, and stop what you are doing. Observe a few minutes of calm, without disturbance, whether you are sitting or lying still or slowly moving around. Let time pass you by, without worry. Just relax and appreciate the moment.

Exercise No. 4 : Chanting a Mantra

A mantra is a short, simple sentence. This exercise could almost be used as a defusion technique, but it is too gentle in the midst of an attack.

Again, it is a form of meditation.

Repeat one or more mantras. This could consist of a set of affirmations. It allows you to see things in a different light, and helps you to get in touch with your inner wisdom. In this case, choose mantras that help you look on the bright side of things and help you calm down when your anxiety levels are on the rise.

For a few minutes, softly and calmly immerse yourself in the mantra and integrate it into your life.

The following are a few examples of mantras, but do not hesitate to make up some of your own :

- "Everything is just fine."

- "I am happy and healthy."

- "I appreciate the moment."

- "When times are tough, I just laugh it off. Things aren't so bad."

- "I feel a bit anxious, but I know it will get better soon."

- "This feeling will pass."

- "I feel good."

These phrases may seem silly to you, but don't worry, you only need to say them in your head. No one needs to know. And you will feel better for doing it, which is the important thing.

Exercise No. 5 : Get out of your Comfort Zone

Perhaps you've been avoiding certain activities because of a fear of having a panic attack while doing them. If this is the case, you need to know that it's important to break out of this vicious circle.

Fear of leaving your home is disabling; your self-confidence plummets, your level of anxiety rises and panic attacks occur more frequently. Therefore, **get out of your comfort zone**. Little by little, try to re-engage in the activities you've been avoiding or dare to try out some new ones.

To get back on track, make a list of things that you would do well if your panic attacks were to suddenly vanish. Think outside the box; do not stop at three activities; you can surely think of ten or more.

Then, rank these activities; start with the one you find the easiest and work your way up to the one that seems the most challenging.

Finally, start reintegrating these activities into your life, little by little. Take note of your successes. Don't let any failures stop you – just try again.

For example, the start of a list could be as follows :

- Enter a crowded store.

- Go out to a restaurant with a group that includes some people you don't know.

- Take an airplane flight.

- Sing to karaoke in public.

...

To successfully re-engage in all your activities, **imagine the worst-case scenario**. Then, dare to try it anyway ! You will find that the worst didn't happen, far from it. You then start to gain a bit of self-confidence and this will help you take back your life.

Next, try exposing yourself to unfamiliar and uncomfortable situations in order to stimulate your self-confidence as well as combat your tendency to get anxious over nothing.

This exercise can easily take over twelve months. Ensure that you have small victories as this will help you maintain your progress. Above all, don't stop trying new things even if an attack was triggered while facing an unfamiliar situation.

Your 'normal' and calmer life will begin as this exercise progresses (In the best-case scenario, progress can happen within months).

Exercise No. 6 : Rationalize your Overall Anxiety

In order to reduce your overall anxiety, make a list of those things which you find overwhelming. Do not confuse this exercise with the previous one in which the goal was to help you rediscover activities that fear of a panic attack caused you to abandon. This time, we are dealing with things that actually worry you. It could be your finances, your children, your parents, your health, your job, a new project...

Write down the source of these problems on a sheet of paper and describe the worst that could happen. I know this part of the exercise is quite unpleasant. Then, once you have written down the worst possible outcome for each situation, give each one a rating from one to ten based on the probability of it actually occurring. This rating will be very subjective, but overall, you'll be forced to admit that some of your worries are not that likely to happen.

It might be interesting to ask someone close to you to share their opinion on the probability of these events occurring. In fact, it is quite likely that you've been exaggerating a bit, a reflex that is quite normal and only human.

Finally, remember to see the glass half-full rather than half-empty. Don't dwell on your problems and the negative side of things. You'll find that life seems a lot easier.

Exercise No. 7 : Make Time for Free Anxiety

This exercise consists of scheduling a time slot, at the same time every day, during which you allow yourself to let your anxious thoughts run free. Take about twenty minutes and express all your worries. Don't do this just before bedtime as you won't sleep well, and you need to ensure you get enough sleep as we saw in the chapter on improving your lifestyle. Instead, choose a time around midday, perhaps during your lunch hour, or after you've finished work, but before the evening.

Now, for the rest of the day, **apart from this time slot, you must not allow yourself to think about your worries**. If something comes up which troubles you during the day, just make note of it on a sheet of paper. Later, during your scheduled period of free anxiety, you can review this paper and agonize about the situation as much as you want. In the meantime, you're not allowing this issue to worry you, or at least, you're not giving it much attention or importance.

The interesting part of this exercise resides in the fact that you gradually lose the habit of thinking negatively, and you learn to keep your negative thoughts under wraps.

It may arrive that, during your free anxiety time slot, you decide to leave certain things out, as you no longer see them as anything you need to make a fuss over. On these occasions, celebrate your progress in gaining control of your negative thoughts.

Exercise No. 8 : Let Everything Explode

This is based on the same principle as the previous exercise, only more intense. It starts with the principle that fighting against anxiety only reinforces it. You will notice that nowhere in any of the defusion techniques have I asked you to triumph over an attack. It is more a question of avoiding it, defusing it, or, at the worst, derailing it.

Now, this time, instead of battling your anxiety or attempting to defuse it, you welcome it with open arms. This is an exposure technique that serves to **desensitize** you. So that you have a clear understanding of this process, we'll use the example of a woman with a phobia against spiders. When she sees a spider nearby, the phobic person jumps up, screams, and climbs up onto a chair. Now, take her to the zoo to see the tarantulas. She will find it difficult to look at these dirty beasts regardless of the fact that they are securely locked up in the vivarium. At first, she will remain at a safe distance. After a few minutes, maybe more, she will want to look at them more closely, even if only for reassurance that they are not going to attack her. Then, several minutes later, she will approach the vivarium of her own accord. Her brain has come to the realization that there is nothing to fear and it has progressively come out of its red alert stage, even though it still remains vigilant.

At this stage, nothing has been done in terms of desensitization.

Allow the person to examine the tarantulas for a few minutes. While she observes them; her brain is analyzing them; their size, the way they move around, how energetic they are, how quickly they move, how susceptible they are to stimuli, etc. The most fascinating thing to her is the sense of danger. From this point on, when she sees a spider at home, the little beast will be somewhat familiar to her. It will be well-defined, and in terms of risk, it is merely a speck of dust compared to the tarantulas in the vivarium. It is quite unlikely that an average house spider will trigger an alert signal as high as it did before. The alert will no longer be red, but orange. With time and experience, she could one day make it yellow, or even make it disappear entirely.

Now, if she sees a little spider while doing housework, the phobic person will still jump back. However, she won't scream and jump onto the closest chair. She has been desensitized; or **rather her brain has adjusted its response to the situation**.

She still has a long way to go, but overall things have improved.

Back to the subject of panic attacks and daily anxiety, it is not necessarily a specific event that triggers a panic attack. At times it can be the brain's exaggerated response to a given situation. That's where the desensitization technique comes in.

When you feel your level of anxiety rising, find a place where you can be alone, then welcome the anxiety. Let it take over, don't try to fight it, just let everything explode. Shout, punch a pillow, jump like a madman, and have fun doing it! Let loose, allow yourself to just let loose !

Let your emotions come out, exaggerate your anxious thoughts, just let it go !

When your level of anxiety is at its peak, although it may seem counter-intuitive, keep going... it will fall. Your level of anxiety will decrease

This exercise helps to desensitize your brain a bit. But note that it should only be used to deal with increased anxiety levels and not with a full-fledged panic attack. It is a preventative exercise, not a defusing technique.

Exercise No. 9 : Ask Yourself Whether the Problem Can Be Solved

Since you are an anxious person by nature, it is likely that you see problems everywhere. I suggest you work at reducing the number of problems that affect you. To do this, ask yourself if this particular problem has a solution, and if there is something you can do about it.

When a worry manifests itself, ask yourself whether it is something that is within your power to resolve.

To do this, ask yourself the following questions :

- Is this a real problem or does it only exist in your mind ?

- If it is imaginary, how likely is it that it will actually happen ?

- What can you do to prepare for it, or is there nothing you can do ?

- If the problem is real, what steps can you take to resolve it ?

If the problem really exists, and you can do something to fix it, don't wait, do it ! After that, you no longer have the problem. Be wary of finding other, fake problems while searching for a solution to the initial problem. Even if the solution is not perfect, you have at least tried to do something to resolve the problem. Then, **take action**, this will relieve the anxiety generated by this worry.

In any other case (you believe the problem has no solution or is imaginary), it is not really a problem for you since there's nothing you can do about it or it doesn't even exist. Dwelling on thoughts such as these is toxic for your mind. Forget about them, and think about something more pleasant. Based on your answers to the previous questions, you can't do anything about it anyway.

For example : You are riding in a car which is traveling on a narrow road beside a river. Since you are not the driver, it's pointless for you to worry about falling into this river. Just trust the driver and don't think about it again.

Another example : You leave for the theater a bit late and start worrying that by the time you arrive, all the seats will be sold out. So, you start berating yourself and putting yourself down because you didn't reserve seats ahead of time. However, you are already waiting in line. The fact that you may not get a seat is beyond your control. Don't waste your time fretting over it, and instead try to think of a Plan B if need be, such as taking in a movie instead. Then, the following week just organize things a bit better.

Exercise No. 10 : Watch a Comedy

Watching funny movies, plays or sketches are all excellent ways to reduce your daily anxiety. Why ? Because they make you laugh. The act of laughing causes the secretion of a pleasure hormone that puts you in a good mood.

Obviously, only one comedy a month will not help much. As with training for sports, watching comedy shows on a regular basis offers better results. Therefore, plan to watch several humorous shows a week.

Participating in recreational activities with friends or family will also bring you pleasure and contribute to your overall well-being, so try to do this as much as possible.

Exercise No. 11 : Keep a Private Journal

Every evening, take a moment to write down what's on your mind in your journal. Don't look for problems; just take note of what comes to mind. Then, analyze these issues by putting all the sources of anxiety that you have identified into perspective.

Play an active part in your progress. For example, this evening you can say that you've decided to keep a daily journal to help reduce your anxiety.

The same holds true for your problems. Don't allow them to get out of hand. Take control. To do this : identify your problems, take a step back from them, and then take action. This will have the effect of reducing their intensity, perhaps even causing them to disappear completely. Make note of the steps you took in your journal.

When in doubt, writing in your personal journal helps you see more clearly, thus allowing you to regain your smile and sense of calm.

Exercise No. 12 : Choose the Things You Wish to See

In the first part of this book, I advised you to see the glass half-full instead of half-empty. The main idea here is to have a more positive and productive state of mind. One way to help with this is by reducing the amount of negative information and increasing the amount of positive information that your mind filters through each day. There are many publications or websites which list positive affirmations. And you don't need to focus on all the unhappiness in the world that you hear about every day in the news.

In order to live a more serene life, choose sources of positive information and surround yourself with positive individuals. This helps reduce the daily anxiety that is felt when brooding about future uncertainty and all the misfortunes that occur every day. It's possible for good things to happen as well. Ask around. Look for the good news.

Exercise No. 13 : Make Love More Often

Falling under the category of "perfectly pleasant physical activity", as well as a powerful source of pleasure; there is nothing better than sexual intercourse. You feel better after sex because hormones of happiness and love bring you peace of mind. Therefore, if you have the good fortune to share your life with a significant other, increase the frequency of your relations (with their consent, of course). This will do wonders for your well-being, and that of your partner as well.

Exercise No. 14 : Make a Clean Sweep

Sometimes, your anxiety level stays high because of the environment in which you spend the bulk of your time. Your surroundings can have a big impact on your state of mind. Simplify your life in order to reduce your anxiety levels on an everyday basis. To do this you can :

- Get rid of all the clutter. At home, pick up all the clothes that are laying around, the stacks of magazines that are waiting to be organized or thrown out, all the miscellaneous junk sitting on the table that doesn't belong there, all of this detracts from your peace of mind, and increases your level of anxiety on a daily basis. Do the same at work, organize your files or tools to avoid wasting 10 minutes of your time searching for something that, if it were in its proper place, would only take a matter of seconds to find. It may seem simple, but it does help reduce your anxiety level. However, don't go to the other extreme and become obsessive about it.

- Redecorate a room or two, your living room for example. Paint the walls, get new cushions, reupholster the couch, change the layout of the furniture, get new knick-knacks, change the photos or paintings on the walls. Giving your surroundings a new look helps you escape your daily routine.

- Change your habits. Wander around in a different park, visit new places, change your weekend routine, take a different route to and from work. Doing this stimulates your brain and has a positive effect on your habits. Even people who tend to stay home most of the time are pleasantly pleased after a new experience.

Exercise No. 15 : Go for a Walk in the Woods

Studies have shown that walking in the forest for more than twenty minutes has a positive effect on anxiety levels. Personally, I am a great fan of a stroll in the forest; it's no problem for me to make it last an hour or two. It seems that this natural environment with its smells and sounds calms the brain. We are well aware that birdsong is known to reduce claustrophobia-related anxiety. So, go out and find it at the source, in the forest. And finally, it's a great opportunity to mull over different issues that may be on your mind or take stock of the progress you have made.

Exercise No. 16 : So, Then ? How About that Half-full Glass ?

Keep in mind that most of the time everything is going well. We can't truthfully tell ourselves that everything that happens is "always" wrong. Take notice of the moments when everything is fine. These are the moments where you're not focusing on your anxiety symptoms. You'll find that they often correspond to periods of time when you were busy on some project and therefore not focusing on yourself. And notice that these moments occur far more often than you think.

Hold on to these thoughts, throughout your day. It will help you avoid dramatizing.

2.2.B-LIFESTYLE CHANGES

In addition to integrating a few exercises to your daily routine to help reduce the anxiety you feel in the present moment, it is important to change a few bad lifestyle habits. In effect, our anxiety level is controlled by the levels of hormones in our brain, and these can be balanced through sane lifestyle choices.

My first recommendation is to **minimize the consumption of stimulants** such as : alcohol, drugs, coffee, tea, soft drinks and tobacco.

These substances promote the occurrence of anxiety attacks. Therefore, the more you reduce your consumption, the better, at least until your panic attacks go away.

Regarding the relaxation effect that drinking alcoholic beverages is supposed to bring, be aware that these effects last only as long as there's alcohol in your system. Your level of anxiety will rise even higher than it was before you took that drink once the alcohol in your blood starts to decrease. It takes somewhat longer for the psychotropic effects of alcohol consumption to diminish.

As for cigarette smoking, studies have shown that it only serves to aggravate nervous tension and anxiety due to poor oxygenation and an increase of toxins in the blood; the exact opposite of what a smoker believes when he says he needs a cigarette to calm down. This feeling of calm is on account of the end of nicotine withdrawal, but is reversed by the secondary effects mentioned above. What actually calms the smoker is not contained within the cigarette itself but in the act of going out for a smoke or simply lighting up. (change of context).

The second recommendation which will have a strong effect on your hormonal balance is **the practice of regular aerobic exercise** for at least thirty minutes.

Exercising only once per week is too little, aim for at least three times per week.

Being active for less than twenty minutes per session is not enough to strongly reduce your anxiety levels. To gain significant benefits from an exercise program, you need to do sessions of at least thirty minutes.

Start slowly, with gentle stretches to warm up, and then gradually increase the intensity of the movement until you reach maximum lung capacity, a period of about fifteen minutes. This is done to avoid injury, which would put an end to your initiative, and that would be very unfortunate.

An aerobic activity is any activity that increases oxygen consumption through deep breathing to the point that you feel out of breath. A leisurely walk is not an aerobic activity even if it lasts for two hours and your legs hurt afterwards. Race walking, running, jogging, swimming and cycling are all aerobic activities and require only a small investment to start.

Exercise has an enormous effect on your general anxiety levels and reduces the number of panic attacks. Therefore, if you don't like sports, it may be time to change your point of view. And, if you feel you don't have enough time during the week, you need to reorganize your schedule and make time. You need to make it a priority, it's that important !

The third recommendation I have for you is also very effective. **Learn how to meditate**. There are many different meditation techniques, as well as a large number of books on the subject. Learn more about this practice, and make it a part of your daily routine. It will go a long way towards limiting or even interrupting a panic attack.

In a nutshell, meditation consists of freeing your mind from all thoughts. It can be practiced in a non-religious context. The act of meditating is to focus on the present moment and/or to concentrate on a reference point, in an effort to rein in the wandering, chattering mind. With practice, you will be able to empty your mind, focus on what is important, relax, remain lucid, and benefit from thousands of other psychological and physiological benefits confirmed by modern science. I am a scientifically-trained atheist, so believe me when I say meditation is not magic, but merely an efficient practice to increase well-being. I strongly encourage you to learn more about this topic if you haven't already done so.

The fourth recommendation is to make sure you get **adequate sleep**. It is absolutely imperative that you get enough sleep every night. If this isn't possible, then take a power nap for fifteen to twenty minutes (but no more) during the day. Don't try to catch up on lost sleep by sleeping in on Sunday as it's not as effective for hormone synthesis. After a poor night's sleep, you are more nervous and more anxious, which, in turn, increases the risk of a panic attack. This is normal - your body is in "defense" mode because it knows it has to operate at a diminished capacity. The same holds true if you slept a sufficient number of hours but the sleep was of poor quality. This may be the case, for example, if you went to bed while under the influence of alcohol or if your night was interrupted several times. Take whatever means necessary to remain undisturbed while you sleep.

I strongly suggest that you do not limit yourself to following just one of these recommendations. It is the combined effect of all these suggestions that will bring about the greatest benefit. Reducing or eliminating stimulants, taking up an aerobic activity, meditating and getting a good night's sleep are really the bare minimum as far as new habits that must be incorporated into your lifestyle in order to reduce the number of panic attacks.

If you succeeded in reducing the frequency of your

anxiety attacks in the past, and are now experiencing a relapse, ask yourself if you have not slipped back into those old, unhealthy habits. This could explain the relapse, or at least help you get back on the right track.

There are other recommendations that may improve your condition. Their effect on your anxiety levels is not as profound as with the previous ones, but they should be considered as well.

Have a healthy diet. Reduce or eliminate your consumption of processed and fast foods, while increasing your intake of fruits and vegetables. Having a balanced diet is extremely important. Don't shortchange yourself by not eating meat, it is essential for getting the iron you need for proper oxygenation of your organs, including the brain. Don't skimp on eating starchy foods under the pretext that you're on a diet; they are needed for energy, and your brain uses a lot of it. Eating a variety of fruits and vegetables (make sure to get an assortment of colors) provides the vitamins and minerals needed to enhance your physiological well-being as well as your mental alertness.

Get some sun; it helps your body synthesize certain elements necessary to your well-being. It's a form of phototherapy, or light therapy. Perhaps you count among the thirty per cent of the population that is sensitive to sunlight (like me). In that case, when you have a choice between drinking an orange juice indoors and taking it outside to the terrace such that you can catch a few rays of sunshine, don't hesitate, it will do you a world of good.

Manage your time to incorporate moments of pleasure. It is important to feel good. If you do not have time for the small pleasures of life, it means you need to reorganize your schedule and make time.

When it comes to small moments of pleasure, a nice, hot bath can be very soothing. By adding a few drops of lavender essential oil, you also get the benefits of a plant used for its soothing virtues for millennia.

As for the rest, don't think that you will relieve your panic attacks with what follows. This is but a grain of sand in the ocean of worries that you may have. However, if you're reducing or eliminating stimulants then you may as well substitute more soothing substances. Here is a small assortment to consume as an infusion or in the form of a pill :

chamomile, marigold flower, magnolia, licorice, parsley, garlic, passion flower, horehound, orange blossom, and valerian root. This last ingredient has an unusual scent but produces undeniable effects on anxiety as it binds to the same receptors as do certain drugs that may be prescribed to reduce anxiety. It is definitely the most powerful element of the mix.

The third and final part of this book looks at a case study in which various defusion techniques are applied during the course of a panic attack.

PART 3:
CASE STUDY

In this section, I will describe an unpleasant experience : the occurrence of a panic attack during a business meeting based on an actual experience.

I will use the first person singular in this scenario. Read through it as if it were happening to you. It is important to make the effort to visualize both the scene AND the implementation of the defusion technique used at each stage of the process. In this way, you will be better prepared should you find yourself in a similar situation.

The narration (in italics) is interspersed with an analysis of the situation as the scene unfolds. You will notice that any moment can correspond to a particular technique. That is why it is best to be comfortable with multiple techniques from the list given in the previous chapter.

Obviously, your experience will differ when it comes down to the fine details but generally most panic attacks have the same general progression which consists of this sequence : apprehension, the first symptoms, onset of the attack, its climax and its aftermath. Don't hesitate to use the techniques that are the best fit for you.

Onset of a panic attack during a business meeting :

It's a gloomy day of a rather chilly autumn. Not motivating at all. Add to this the fact that I have a business meeting late in the morning. Even before the time of the meeting, I start to feel anxious. I often feel uncomfortable at these meetings as I never know what new responsibilities I'll get stuck with. In addition, there's a chance I'll be reprimanded for being behind schedule in my current tasks. The whole situation paints a pretty bleak picture. Nevertheless, "When you gotta go, you gotta go !"

I hadn't even entered the room yet but the temperature already felt more like summer. Is it me ? Did somebody turn off the air conditioning ? I don't even bother to ask a colleague, it has to be me, of course.

We see here that my anticipation anxiety begins to manifest early on. I start to weaken even before I enter the room. Furthermore, I focus on myself rather than trying to reconnect with the exterior, i.e. with the people around me and the place where I am. As I head towards the conference room, I should be practicing deep breathing or even full breathing techniques. Adding in a few muscle tensions/ relaxations with my fists and forearms would also be helpful, as would conversing with colleagues who are also on their way to the meeting as this would help me reconnect with the outside world.

However, I am unaware of these techniques, so I do nothing special. On the contrary, I keep worrying.

All is well for the moment. It is normal to be nervous about certain events ... to some extent.

I arrive at the conference room on time and our supervisor invites us to enter. Without giving it much thought, I enter mechanically, head bowed, and make a beeline for the back of the room. This means I'll be as far from the door as possible, with others impeding the way to the exit. Naturally, the air conditioner blowing out cool air is right next to the door.

The meeting begins, led by our supervisor. We will speak in turn to comment on various topics and share our points of view. There are three people who are likely to speak before me, meaning a long wait before my turn comes. The room feels even hotter. Moreover, I find the meeting room very small and confined for the number of people present. Confusion takes over, my mouth is dry and I feel as if I have something stuck in my throat.

As expected, my anxiety has not abated one bit, on the contrary, I feel even more uncomfortable. I haven't chosen the best seat and I feel like a prisoner where I am. Of course, despite the mandatory nature of this meeting, I am not a prisoner. I remain a free adult with liberty of action (important information for the rest of the scene). This feeling of imprisonment develops in my imagination because of my sub-optimal position in the room and the intimidating presence of my superior.

In retrospect, upon entering the room, I should have taken a seat near the door (less anxiety provoking and more practical should I need to leave quickly). In addition, I would have had the added benefit of the cooler air from the air conditioner, which might have helped reduce this choking sensation. Having visual access to the outside could also help reduce anxiety. Had there been a window in this conference room, it would have been better to face it rather than turn my back to it and face the wall. Also, I should have gotten a glass of water to avoid this dry mouth and ease the discomfort in my throat.

Once again, I don't focus on the discussion around me but on my hypothetical, perhaps even imaginary, symptoms.

For the moment, all is still well. I'm managing the situation, and soon it will be my turn to speak.

It's my turn. Our leader reiterates the question, turning towards me. Surely he must have noticed that my mind was elsewhere. His gaze strikes me as oppressive. For better or for worse, I manage to stammer the speech I had prepared in advance. He asks for more details, but it quickly becomes apparent to him that I don't have much to say today. He must think I'm not very helpful or just plain stupid. It's in my best interest to do a better job next time. He turns and moves on to the next speaker.

Discreetly, I breathe a sigh of relief. This exhale is certainly the only moment of relaxation at this meeting. It's stifling in this room. However, at least one of us is allowed to crack a few jokes. Or rather, I suppose his remarks were funny as the others chuckled a few times.

The moment of greatest distraction to the brain just occurred, namely, having to answer a question that was put directly to me. Now, I am again left to my own devices, mulling over these negative thoughts about my poor response and the possible consequences to my career in the short term, or so I think. I'd be better off listening to the other speakers, then, I'd learn that their answers are no better than mine.

In addition, I am still completely closed off to external events such as funny turns of phrase, for example. I focus too much on the symptoms that flared up after my performance. Instead, I should be quick to use techniques such as "stop and replace", the "cheat sheet", "controlled or full breathing", or "find a distraction".

The "stop and replace" technique would be an appropriate tool to battle the negative ruminations that come to mind regarding my 'poor' performance and what my boss thinks of my usefulness or efficiency. After all, the dissatisfaction he seems to express is more likely due to the fact that he can't decide which action to take based on the responses he has received so far. And he doesn't see an easy way out. Therefore, he is worried about making the wrong decision. He is human, after all. So, viewed from that perspective, he most likely hasn't given my performance much thought at all.

The 'cheat sheet' is another technique that could be used here. Once attention is no longer focused on me, I read my 'cheat sheet' and see : "Could I be exaggerating the situation ?" or "It's just a difficult time, it will not last forever." This would allow me to put the situation into perspective and stop being anxious for no good reason. I could even go so far as to take pleasure in seeing the tense expression on my colleague's face (the one I do not like) as he struggles to say his piece. (This would probably distract me because I really don't like him ... however, it's not nice to wish misfortune on others, right ?)

Somewhat less intellectual, more active, and without wishing ill on my colleague, I could practice controlled breathing, discreetly, so no one will notice. Nevertheless, I need to keep my brain active to occupy my mind. To do this, I could focus on successfully performing the controlled breathing technique, an essential element for it to be effective.

I could distract my brain by listening to the jokes and what others are saying. I could also review my previous answer and think about how I could provide more detail and make it more relevant before we move on to another subject.

Alas, I do none of this. The situation goes from bad to worse.

Gradually, nausea overtakes me. I choke, or at least I feel as though I am. I look at the others with a barely concealed look of worry. I get the impression they realize that I'm going to faint, but they're trying to hide it. Dizziness is intense, I feel a flush of sweat on my forehead and I can no longer hold onto my pen. I feel as if all the strength has drained out of me.

The panic attack is clearly underway. At this stage, it takes a massive amount of will to conceal my state from others. At this point, the best would have been for one of my colleagues in the room, in whom I have great confidence and get on well with, to come to my aid and comfort me. As we saw in the previous chapter, he could have been a positive influence and kept me from 'blowing sky high.'

Unfortunately, this was not the case. The upward spiral is engaged.

I don't feel well at all. To the point that I cannot or don't care to hide it, assuming that others are still oblivious to what's going on. My vision becomes blurry; I no longer have the strength to raise my hand to signal. I feel like I'm going to die, right here, right now, with no one showing the least bit of concern, in the conference room closest to my workstation, one gloomy autumn morning.

Remember, the feeling that you are going to die is only an illusion. Moreover, the attack will subside and eventually stop, and you will survive. Thank goodness ! But, when you're right in the midst of it, and barely lucid, you think it's too late and there's nothing you can do. And it's at this moment, when the crisis is at its worst that you must say : 'No, never !'

I have told you many times that you should never attempt to fight a growing panic attack. But once the crisis is at its peak, it's a different story, with the possible exception of attacks coupled with hyperventilation; a phenomenon which I, personally, have never experienced.

Those who have suffered many panic attacks in the past can learn to recognize the apex easily; it is generally that point at which you imagine that you're going to die on the spot, without moving a muscle, although you could still move if you came back to your senses.

Once you arrive at a point where, in practice, things cannot get any worse, it's time to take control. And having a strong will could help you greatly.

At that critical moment when you say, "I'm going to die !" you respond simply and in a very firm tone, "No. This is not true." Repeat it if necessary (and it surely will be). Later, when your reason manifests, take the opportunity to remind yourself that the right questions are listed on your cheat sheet. Answer them one by one, and be honest, without painting an overly bleak picture of the situation.

In the worst-case scenario, change your surroundings. This is likely to be what you will do anyway. Simply changing your thoughts (e.g. thinking of the evening you have planned with friends tonight) is not powerful enough at this point. You need to physically get out of the room. And, from the moment you step out into the corridor and hear the door close the behind you, you begin to feel a whole lot better. Well, at least you won't feel quite as bad.

To help you calm down faster, make use of the "go for a change of scene", "seek solace", or "engage in physical activity" techniques.

Changing your surroundings will completely change the game for your brain, which is good for regaining control of the situation. In addition, it will facilitate the application of the following techniques.

Seek comfort from a colleague outside the meeting room. Together, step outside for some fresh air, or find a private spot where you can talk about what happened and be comforted by your colleague without worrying about the curious stares of others.

Engage in physical activity, by finding another conference room or leaving the building to walk for a while and find a private place where you can let off some steam.

After all, you had to leave the meeting because of this panic attack, so be sure to take the time to get it right and do whatever it takes to regain your composure.

After this interlude which was directly addressed to you, let's get back to my story and its ending.

In a last ditch effort, I left the room claiming a sudden urge to go without elaborating as to why. And I went outside to get some air, taking the stairs instead of the elevator. This was no time to get stuck with someone in a metal cage for the time it takes to go down three floors. A few minutes pass. I walk for a bit in the fresh air. Finally, this chilly autumn is good for something. I feel better now. But the meeting is not over yet. Should I go back? I don't know…Time passes. The longer I stay away, the more implausible my pretext of an unexpected phone call becomes. And slowly but surely, my anxiety starts to creep up again. This is a fine kettle of fish I've gotten myself into! What do I tell them now? Stop thinking and do something! I'll make my way back to the conference room, taking my time, hoping to keep my composure. But I don't know if I can handle going back into that room.

Should I go back? This depends on, first of all, whether I have regained my composure, and secondly, whether I am now convinced that the panic attack was triggered for no real reason, i.e. **it was only a disproportionate response of my brain to a danger that does not even exist**. If these two things are clear to me, there is no reason for me not to go back, as not doing so would only add fuel to the next crisis. If, on the contrary, things are not so obvious to me, then maybe I'd better wait it out while trying to regain some sense of composure.

After a fair amount of procrastination, I decide to go back into the meeting room. However, the meeting had already broken up. I am ashamed and afraid to explain what happened. Fortunately, my colleagues are happy to get out of the meeting; they are in good spirits and tease me about all the time I took. Without saying a word, I smile.

Things turned out all right this time (relatively speaking). But it is obvious that I'd better learn to manage my shame and my fear of having to explain or justify myself. It would have been a good move to continue practicing deep breathing to calm myself and gain more insight into this emotional roller-coaster ride that hijacked my morning.

What a day ! I'm sure you can relate…

A panic attack, such as the one described above, could happen in other more or less anxiety-provoking situations. It's up to you to make use of the information in this anecdote to better handle your own anxiety. Learn to incorporate the various defusion techniques into your daily life so that you are better equipped to use them should the need arise as this could be a great help in managing a future panic attack.

In any case, if you feel as if an attack will occur, it most likely will. Should this be the case, don't fight it; don't complain about it. Just accept the situation and deal with it. This is the best way to ensure that everything turns out for the best, or at worst, the least possible harm.

I chose to describe the onset of a panic attack at a business meeting. It could also have occurred in a personal or job interview, during a romantic encounter, at the wheel of a car, or in the middle of the night while alone in bed. While these situations may occur, do not try to avoid them at all costs as by repeating your exposure to them they become less anxiety-provoking. In any case, you will not die (However, if you're driving, consider pulling over to make sure you really won't. But that goes without saying, right ?). Face your demons; you will only come out stronger. You learn from every experience, whether it is good or bad. The very act of avoiding new experiences makes you more vulnerable. So, dare to move forward and give yourself the proper tools and techniques to eliminate your anxiety attacks once and for all. It's possible, I did it. And I know I'm not the only one. You can, too. It's up to you.

CONCLUSION

Anxiety attacks are not inevitable. Apart from very serious cases where it is best to consult a professional, it is entirely possible to live without them and have a more peaceful life. To reach this point, you must take yourself in hand, accept this momentary challenge, and take the necessary steps to prevent future relapses.

In this sense, I hope that this book has provided you with invaluable and practical information which will help you circumvent an emerging panic attack and that, in the future, you will no longer be so negatively affected by anxiety-provoking situations. Of course, I'm assuming that you are applying the techniques and exercises in this book in order to arrive at some noticeable improvements.

Feel free to come back to this book on preventive exercises when you feel you are at a delicate stage of your life. And keep practicing these new and better lifestyle habits to avoid slipping back into a phase where you're experiencing frequent bouts of anxiety and panic attacks.

Take yourself in hand when you find yourself consistently looking at that half-empty glass; there are so many more positive approaches. It's simply a way of looking at things, this tendency of always expecting the worst. Learn to direct your negative thoughts towards more positive ones. And the icing on the cake, the people around you will appreciate your newfound sense of well-being.

Dare to come out of your shell. Every new experience will increase your self-confidence, and will divert any feelings of anxiety you may be experiencing. That which does not kill us makes us stronger. You know all this; just give it some thought when doubt shows its face.

I hope that after reading this book you will be able to live a more 'normal' life, with all its joys and sorrows, but without that ball in the pit of your stomach or that overwhelming feeling of suffocation that overtakes you when there's nothing wrong. Anxiety is not a train that runs over you and crushes the life out of you; it is merely something that must be endured, either alone or in the company of others. If it is good, enjoy it, if not, grin and bear it, but don't worry, everyone will come out alive. :)

THANK YOU

Thank you, dear reader, for taking the time to read this book.

I thank you even more if you would take a couple of minutes to leave a comment or review on the site from which you downloaded this book with the reason why you like it.

If you think this book could be useful to others, let them know about it. They will certainly be grateful to know of its existence. Thanks to you, they will avoid many unfortunate experiences and start enjoying a more pleasant life.

To be informed of the release of new books from me, please register by clicking on the following link: http://brioud.com/sqz-eng-axt.html

Sincerely Yours.

ABOUT THE AUTHOR

Philippe Brioud, a 47-year-old mechanical engineer, used to suffer from extreme anxiety and repeated panic attacks. Problems began after several marital and family difficulties occurred in less than a year. That was a life-changing year for Philippe. Panic attacks came, one after another, for a period of about two years.

After these two years, he finally decides to get his act together.

Now, free of attacks, he understands the problem, how to overcome it and how to avoid a possible relapse.

In his book, "How to Ease Anxiety and Panic Attacks and Free Yourself from Them", Philippe shares the psychological tools and techniques he has learned and which he knows are effective.

It's up to you to take yourself in hand so that you, in turn, can enjoy a more peaceful life.